Superfoods

Matcha Green Tea, Learn the Miraculous Benefits of the Matcha Superfood and Tons of Great Matcha Recipes

Ariana Hunter

© 2015

Disclaimer / Copyright Info

Introduction

Matcha Green Tea is a finely ground, or fine powder green tea. Matcha is used in Japan for ceremonial purposes such as serving, preparation, and drinking. Today, Matcha is used as a food dye and natural sweetener.

The skin care products, and hair care products that you find in your favorite department store, grocery store, or gas station, contain many harmful chemicals that will contaminate your body and irritate your skin.

To make it worse, these products are produced by companies that have no concern for your health. These companies are looking out for their wallets, and exercise no discretion when choosing the ingredients they decide to dump into these products. This is alarming because consumers are not aware of the harmful effects of these horrifying ingredients.

Another harsh reality is that the FDA has not set any restrictions on the use of these nasty and harmful ingredients. Sadly, this only encourages consumers to go out and stock up on these deadly products.

This book contains valuable information on Matcha Green Tea. That will come later. For now let's look at some of the many benefits of this tasty superfood.

Chapter 1 – Benefits of Matcha

Fight Cancer with Matcha

The antioxidants in Matcha Green Tea are very powerful. They are so powerful that they have the potency to aid your body in fighting off cancer. One particular antioxidant is catechin EGCg (epigallocatechin gallate). Catechin has the ability to slow down the growth of fatal cancer cells, and can stop cancer cells from forming. One cup of Matcha Green Tea has 137 times the amount of catechin, than your regular, overestimated green tea. So, Matcha Green Tea is definitely something you should have in your possession at all times.

Energy Increaser

Matcha has the ability to increase your energy and caffeine has nothing to do with it. The natural composition of Matcha can also improve stamina by up 30%. So, if you are low on energy, and need an extra boost of energy. You should look to Matcha green tea to save the day!

Weight Loss

Matcha green tea will be a great addition to your diet if you are looking to lose weight or just simply maintain a healthy weight. Matcha is a super metabolism booster and the ultimate fat burner. Studies have shown that Matcha helps burn calories up to four time faster, and does not put extra stress on the body. It will not raise the heart rate or blood pressure, which makes it one of the best solutions for those looking to lose weight.

The Go-to for Detoxification

Matcha is rich in Chlorophyll which means that it is rich in antioxidants. It gets its overabundance in Chlorophyll from the fact that it is grown in the shade. Matcha will rid the body of heavy metals, nasty toxins, and harmful chemicals. With extremely powerful anti-bacterial and antioxidant properties, Matcha green tea is also a good source of blood cleaning chlorophyll.

The Hair Grower

Matcha green tea is rich in Panthenol. Most of the hair care products on the market contain Panthenol due to its unrefuted ability repair split ends and stimulate hair growth. You can receive benefits of this hair stretching vitamin by either drinking Matcha green tea or applying the tea directly to your scalp. This will dramatically strengthen your hair.

Skin Care

High Fiber beans, veggies, and raw fruits contain high levels of antioxidants. In comparison to these foods, Matcha green tea trumps all when it comes to antioxidants. This is great because it has the ability to improve the appearance of your skin and slow down the aging process.

We hope you enjoy drinking green tea as much as you'll enjoy eating it, applying is to your skin, and hair.

Chapter 2 – History of Matcha

Green tea originated in China and has been widely cultivated in Japan for thousands of years. It has become very popular in America and is now one of the most admired beverages in Japan. However, green tea used to be so scarce and so cherished that it was only available to select monks.

All of that changed when a 12th century Zen monk by the name of Eisai, presented Matcha to the public, and made this healthy and powerful beverage available for everyone to enjoy. Drinking tea was originally was used for medicinal purposes, but once the health benefits had been discovered, many people became accustomed to adding green tea to their diet.

By the end of the 12th century, green tea began to be prepared using a process called tencha. This procedure consisted of powdered tea and hot water being whipped together in a bowl. This process carried on to the 13th where it was adopted by Samurais, where they incorporated it into ceremonial practices.

The Japanese tea ceremony begins with the host properly cleaning the tea bowl, the tea scoop, and the tea whisk with concentrated and graceful movement. Once the utensils are cleaned, three scoops of Matcha powder per guest is added to the bowl. Hot water is ladled into the bowl and the mixture is whisked into a thin paste. More water is added as needed to create a soup-like tea. The bowl is offered to the first guest and bows are exchanged before the guest admires the bowl, rotates it, and then sips. The guest wipes the bowl and presents it to the next guest who repeats these movements. Once the final guest has sipped, the bowl is returned to the host who will rinse and clean the tea whisk and scoop again.

Finally, by the 16th century, tea drinking had spread to all levels of society in Japan and became a forte in Japanese culture. And today many are becoming accustomed to using Matcha as a beverage that can bring them many health benefits and seemingly magical cures.

Chapter 3 – Ingestion is the BEST WAY!

Nature never lets us down. It has provided us with the perfect ingredients for the perfect health. The great thing about Matcha Green Tea is that it is cost efficient and you can incorporate it in many parts of your daily regimen. Consuming Matcha green tea produces the best results.

Matcha Tips

- To avoid Matcha tasting bitter, do not add Matcha to boiling water.
- A Bamboo whisk is the best utensil to use to mix.
- Matcha should be stored in the freezer in order to maintain freshness and enhance the sweetness. When ready to use, allow Matcha to adjust to room temperature before using.
- It is recommended to soften up your Bamboo whisk before you begin to make your Matcha. You can soften your whisk by simply dipping it in hot water.
- Add Matcha green tea to your diet in order to make detox a breeze. The chlorophyll in Matcha assists our bodies in removing heavy

metals and chemicals from the bloodstream and the rest of our organs.

- Great coffee replacement!
- Make any dish a lean green machine by adding Matcha. Mix together 1 tablespoon Himalayan Pink Salt and ½ tsp Matcha Green Tea Powder and sprinkle it over the top. You'll love it!
- Perfect for healthy smoothies and milkshakes
- Fight off colds with Matcha. Matcha green tea contains a large arsenal of Vitamin C, antioxidants, carotenoids, manganese, and tocopherols. These play a HUGE role in help your body fight off nasty viruses and bacteria's.

Here are some amazing recipes that show you how AMAZING and versatile this stuff really is!

Green Brownies

Yield: *Twelve Servings*

Active Time: *15 minutes*

Cooking Time: *25 minutes*

Total Time: *40 minutes*

Ingredients

- ¼ cup organic Matcha Green Tea powder
- ½ cup unpasteurized almonds, toasted
- 2 free-range eggs
- 6 tbsp ghee
- 1 cup unbleached flour
- 6 ounce organic white chocolate bar (30% cacao content), melted
- ½ cup organic white chocolate chips (30% cacao content)
- ½ tsp vanilla bean powder
- ¼ tsp almond extract
- Unrefined Extra Virgin Olive Oil

Cooking Directions

1. Set oven to 350 degrees and lightly grease an 8"x8" baking pan with olive oil. Set to the side.
2. Mix together all ingredients in a large bowl until fully blended.
3. Pour batter into the prepared baking pan. Spread the batter using a spatula to ensure even baking.
4. Bake for a minimum of 20 to 25 minutes or until a toothpick comes out clean when placed in the center of the brownie.
5. Cut into twelve even sections and enjoy!

Matcha Protein Bars

Yield: *Ten Servings*

Active Time: *10 minutes*

Cooking Time: *10 minutes*

Total Time: *20 minutes*

Ingredients

- 4 tsp organic Matcha Green Tea powder
- 8 scoops vanilla brown rice protein powder
- 4 ounces cacao nibs, melted
- ⅓ cup organic roasted almond butter
- 1 cup almond milk
- 1 tbsp organic Agave nectar
- ½ cup oat flour
- 1 tbsp lemon juice, freshly squeezed

Cooking Directions

1. Line an 8"x8" baking pan with olive oil. Set to the side.
2. Beat together almond butter, milk, agave nectar, and lemon juice in a large bowl using an electric hand mixer on low speed. Set to the side.
3. Combine flour, Matcha powder, and protein powder in a medium bowl. Stir until all of the dry ingredients are well blended. Slowly pour dry ingredients into the wet ingredients bowl while beating with the electric hand mixer. Keep mixing until the mixture begins to appear as cookie dough.
4. Scrap the batter into the baking pan and press to flatten and even out. Cover with plastic wrap, and allow to chill in the fridge overnight.

5. When ready to serve, slice into 10 to 12 protein bars. Drizzle with melted cacao and enjoy!

Matcha Pistachio Butter Cups

Yield: *12 Butter Cups*

Active Time: *5 minutes*

Cooking Time: *0 minutes*

Total Time: *5 minutes*

Ingredients

Cup:

- 5 ounces organic white chocolate (30% cacao content), melted
- 1 tsp organic Matcha Green Tea powder

Filling:

- ½ tsp organic Matcha Green Tea powder
- 1 cup pistachios, peeled and rinsed
- 1 tbsp Unrefined Virgin Coconut oil
- 2 tbsp Fondant and Icing (powdered 100% pure can sugar)

Cooking Directions

1. Line a 12 cup mini muffin pan with cupcake wrappers. Set to the side.

For the Filling:

2. Add pistachios into a food processor, and blend for about 15 minutes or until the nuts form into a ball. Be sure to scrap the sides when the nut splatter on the outside of the cup. The final product should resemble peanut butter. Add Matcha Green Tea and blend to combine. Sift fondant icing sugar over the pistachio butter.

Mix well to combine, and form into 12 balls. Each ball should measure to about 1 teaspoon. Set to the side.

Cup:

3. In medium bowl, stir together melted white chocolate and Matcha Green Tea. Mix until well combined. Pour about 1 teaspoon of the chocolate mixture into each lined muffin cup, and smooth the mixture around the sides of the lined muffin cups. Allow to chill in the fridge for a minimum of 15 to 20 minutes.
4. Flatten the pistachio balls before adding them to the hardened white chocolate cups. Top each filled cup with 1 teaspoon of chocolate mixture. Be sure to completely cover the filling. Place in the fridge for a minimum of 1 hour or until the chocolate has set. Enjoy at room temperature.

Smoothie Vanilla Matcha

Yield: *Two Servings*

Active Time: *5 minutes*

Cooking Time: *0 minutes*

Total Time: *5 minutes*

Ingredients

- 2 frozen organic bananas (peel before freezing)
- 1 cup organic almond milk
- 2 tbsp organic Matcha Green Tea powder
- 1 tbsp organic Agave nectar
- 2 tsp vanilla bean powder
- 1 cup spring water ice

Cooking Directions

1. Add all of the ingredients to the blender, and puree until all of the ingredients become completely smooth.
2. Pour into your favorite glass and enjoy!

More Matcha Protein Bars

Yield: One Large Bowl

Active Time: 10 minutes

Cooking Time: 0 minutes

Total Time: 3 hours, 10 minutes

Ingredients

- 1 tsp organic Matcha Green Tea powder
- 1 cup organic almond milk
- 1 tbsp organic rolled oats
- 2 tbsp chia seeds (divided)
- 1 tbsp lemon juice, freshly squeezed
- 2 tbsp organic Agave nectar
- 1 tsp vanilla bean powder

Cooking Directions

1. Add 1 tablespoon of chia seeds and remaining ingredients into a blender. Blend until the ingredients are fully combined, and has reached a creamy consistency.
2. Pour into a medium to large bowl and slowly mix in remaining chia seeds. Set in the fridge to chill for a minimum of 3 hours or until it gels and it reaches a nice pudding consistency.
3. When ready to serve top with a sprinkle of Matcha and desired amount of Agave nectar.

Chocolate Matcha Berry Smoothie

Yield: *Two Servings*

Active Time: *5 minutes*

Cooking Time: *0 minutes*

Total Time: *5 minutes*

Ingredients

- ½ cup fresh strawberries, sliced
- ⅛ cup organic Matcha Green Tea powder
- 5 ounces organic white chocolate (30% cacao content)
- 2 tbsp organic cacao powder
- 2 tbsp organic raw Goji berries
- 1 tsp organic Maca powder
- 1 tbsp organic coconut peanut butter
- 1 cup coconut water
- ¼ avocado, chopped
- 1 tbsp organic Agave nectar
- ⅓ cup plain Greek yogurt
- Spring water ice (optional)

Cooking Directions

1. Add all of the ingredients to the blender, and puree until all of the ingredients become completely smooth.
2. Pour into your favorite glass and enjoy!

Green Banana Cream Nibbles

Yield: *Five servings*

Active Time: *20 minutes*

Cooking Time: *15 minutes*

Total Time: *55 minutes*

Ingredients

Angel Bites:

- 5 egg whites
- ⅓ cup monk fruit sweetener, granulated
- 1 tsp organic Matcha Green Tea powder
- 1 ½ tsp vanilla extract
- 1 pinch Himalayan Pink Salt

Banana Cream Filling:

- 2 tsp organic Matcha Green Tea powder
- ½ cup egg substitute
- 1 cup unsweetened almond milk
- 1 tsp vanilla extract
- 2 tbsp light butter
- 1 tbsp cornstarch
- ¼ cup monk fruit sweetener, granulated
- 1 tsp banana flavor
- 2 bananas, sliced
- 2 tbsp semisweet chocolate chips

Cooking Directions

1. Preheat oven to 350 degrees. Coat a 13"x11" baking sheet with cooking spray and set to the side.

2. In a medium bowl, beat egg whites until frothy using a whisk or electric mixer. Discontinue whipping and dump in sweetener, Matcha, salt, and vanilla. Mix on high speed for about 20 to 30 seconds or until egg white mixture medium-stiff peaks.

3. Dump rounded tbsp of the egg white mixture onto the prepared baking sheet. Bake until firm and golden brown this should take about 10 to 15 minutes. Remove the wafers from the oven and allow to cool.

4. Using a blender, combine sweetener and cornstarch. Pour cornstarch mixture, milk, butter, and vanilla into a small pot, and simmer over medium heat for about 3 to 4 minutes. The mixture should be slightly bubbly.

5. Remove the cornstarch blend from heat and add the banana flavor and Matcha. Mix well and place the cornstarch blend into the fridge to chill until ready for about 20 minutes.

6. Build the angel bites by placing the wafers on serving plate with the bottoms facing up. Top each of the wafers with a banana slice, and a spoonful of filing. Stack another angel bite on top.

7. Garnish with chocolate chips. Add whip cream if desired.

Matcha Berry Sorbet

Yield: *Four Servings*

Active Time: *25 minutes*

Freezing Time: *0 minutes*

Total Time: *5 hours*

Ingredients

- 2 tsp organic Matcha Green Tea powder
- 1 ½ cups raspberries
- 1 ½ cups blueberries
- ½ cup 100% pure cane sugar
- 1 ½ tbsp organic Agave nectar
- ¾ cup water
- 1 tsp rose water

Cooking Directions

1. Bring water and sugar to a boil in a large saucepan. Mix well to cover the sugar with water. Immediately reduce heat and allow the simple syrup to simmer until the sugar is completely dissolved. Remove from heat and set to the side for cooling.
2. Add Matcha, berries, simple syrup, nectar, and rose water to a blender. Blend until the berries reach a smooth consistency.
3. Place colander over a large bowl, and strain the pureed berries into the bowl. Cover the bowl with lid or plastic wrap and place in the fridge to chill for at least 2 hours or overnight.
4. In the meantime, place a large, empty bowl into the freezer to chill.

5. Remove the Matcha berry puree from the fridge and blend for about 30 seconds using an immersion blender. Pour blended berries in an ice cream maker and freeze. Be sure to follow the manufacturer's instructions as close as possible when freezing the Matcha berry puree with the ice cream maker.

6. Dump frozen berry puree into the chilled bowl, and return to freezer to chill for an additional 2 hours.

7. Remove from freezer, and allow to soften in the fridge or at room temperate for a minimum of 15 to 30 minutes before diving in.

Blueberry Matcha Cheesecake Bars

Yield: *Twenty servings*

Active Time: *15 minutes*

Cooking Time: *35 minutes*

Total Time: *50 minutes*

Ingredients

- ¾ cup fresh blueberries
- 2 tsp organic Matcha Green Tea powder
- ¼ cup reduced-sugar apricot preserves
- 1 ¼ cups whole-wheat graham cracker crumbs
- 2 large free-range eggs
- 12 ounces grass-fed cream cheese, softened
- ⅓ cup grass-fed sour cream
- 1 cup monk fruit sweetener (divided)
- ⅓ cup Unrefined Extra Virgin Olive oil
- 2 tsp vanilla bean powder
- 1 tbsp water
- Cooking spray

Cooking Directions

1. Set oven to 350 degrees, and coat an 8"x8" baking dish with cooking spray. Set to the side.
2. Mix together graham cracker crumbs, ¼ cup sweetener, and olive oil. Dump graham cracker blend into prepared baking dish, and press mixture down to form a crust. Be sure the graham cracker crust if firmly packed. Bake mixture in the oven for 5 minutes. Remove from oven and set to the side for cooling.

3. Using an electric mixer, beat together Matcha, cream cheese and remaining sweetener together in a large bowl. Gradually add eggs, sour cream, and vanilla. Continue to beat until cream mixture is smooth. Gently fold in blueberries, and dump mixture onto graham cracker crust. Evenly distribute and spread with spatula.

4. Bake for 30 to 35 minutes, or until firm mixture is set and firm. Remove from oven and cool on a wire rack for 30 minutes. Cover with plastic wrap and place in fridge to chill for 2 hours.

5. When cheesecake is set, combine apricot preserves and water in a small saucepan, and melt preserves over medium heat. Stirring constantly. Spread melted preserves over cheesecake, cut into 12 bars, and serve immediately.

Spicy Apricot Squash Muffins

Yield: *Twelve Mini Muffins*

Active Time: *15 minutes*

Cooking Time: *30 minutes*

Total Time: *1 hour, 15 minutes*

Ingredients

- 2 tsp organic Matcha Green Tea powder
- 1 cup butternut squash, cubed
- ½ cup apricot jam
- ½ cup organic oat bran
- 2 free-range eggs, beaten
- 1 cup free-range light cream
- 1 cup 100% pure cane sugar
- 2 cups unbleached all-purpose flour
- 1 tbsp ground ginger
- 2 tsp aluminum-free baking powder
- ½ tsp aluminum-free baking soda
- Spring Water, as needed
- Cooking spray

Cooking Directions

1. Set oven to 375 degrees, and coat a 12 muffin cup pan with cooking spray. Set to the side.
2. Mix together flour, oat bran, ginger, baking powder, and baking soda in a large bowl.
3. Bring squash to a boil over medium-high heat in a large pot. Immediately reduce heat to medium-low and allow to cook for a minimum of 15 minutes. Remove from heat, drain, and mash. Add cream, Matcha, sugar, flour, and

eggs. Mix until the mixture becomes uniform and smooth. Pour even amount of batter into each muffin cup.

4. Bake for a minimum of 20 minutes or until the muffins are lightly browned. Allow to cool before serving.

Pistachio-Green Chai Muffins

Yield: *Twelve Servings*

Active Time: *10 minutes*

Bake Time: *15 minutes*

Total Time: *30 minutes*

Ingredients

- 2 chai blend tea bags, opened
- 4 tsp organic Matcha Green Tea powder
- ⅓ cup shelled dry-roasted pistachios, chopped
- 1 cup free-range buttermilk
- ¼ cup ghee
- 1 ¾ cups unbleached all-purpose flour
- 1 tsp aluminum-free baking powder
- 1 tsp aluminum-free baking soda
- 1 large free-range egg, lightly beaten
- ½ cup packed brown sugar
- ½ cup Fondant and Icing (powdered 100% pure can sugar)
- 1 ½ tsp vanilla bean powder, divided
- 1 tbsp Spring water
- ¼ tsp Himalayan Pink Salt
- Cooking spray

Cooking Directions

1. Set oven to 375 degrees. Coat a 12 cup muffin pan with cooking spray. Set to the side. Lightly add flour into dry measuring cups, and level them off using a knife. Combine all dry ingredients in a large bowl (excluding powdered sugar, ½ tsp vanilla bean powder, and

pistachios), and stir with a whisk. Make a well in center of mixture.

2. Mix buttermilk, ghee, and egg in a bowl, stirring well with a whisk. Add buttermilk mixture to flour mixture, stirring just until moist.

3. Divide batter evenly among prepared muffin cups. Sprinkle nuts evenly over batter.

4. Bake at 375 degrees for a minimum of 15 minutes or until a toothpick inserted in center comes out clean. Cool for 5 minutes in pan on a wire rack.

5. Mix remaining ½ tsp vanilla bean powder, powdered sugar, and 1 tbsp water, stirring until smooth. Drizzle evenly over muffins.

Matcha Potato Soup

Yield: *Ten Servings*

Active Time: *25 minutes*

Cooking Time: *45 minutes*

Total Time: *70 minutes*

Ingredients

- 1 tbsp organic Matcha Green Tea powder
- 3 large leeks, cleaned, rinsed, and thinly sliced
- 1 large fennel bulb, thinly sliced
- 4 large celery stalks, thinly sliced
- 2 large white potatoes, peeled and cubed
- 3 large white onions, peeled and halved
- 3 garlic cloves, minced
- 8 cups Spring water
- 2 tsp celery seed
- 2 ½ tbsp Italian Seasoning
- 2 tbsp fresh parsley, finely chopped
- 2 tbsp Unrefined Extra Virgin Olive oil
- 1 tbsp Himalayan Pink Salt
- 1 ½ tbsp ground black pepper

Cooking Directions

1. Add olive oil, leeks, celery, fennel, onions, garlic, potatoes, salt, and pepper to a large pot and cook over medium-low heat. Sauté until the onions become slightly transparent and vegetables soften or for a minimum of 10 minutes.

2. Slowly pour and stir in 8 cups of water over the sautéed vegetables, and bring to a boil. Mix in celery seed, Italian Seasoning, parsley, and salt and pepper to taste.

3. Stirring occasionally, cook vegetable mixture over low heat for a minimum of 30 minutes or until the vegetables become tender and the mixture begins to thicken. Serve immediately.

Variations

- To add some creaminess to this soup, add a small amount of half and half with about ½ cup parmesan cheese.
- Blend or puree half of the soup to give the soup and extra thickness

Green Strawberry Meringue Bites

Yield: Forty Servings

Active Time: 15 minutes

Cooking Time: 75 minutes

Total Time: 90 minutes

Ingredients

- 40 organic strawberries
- 2 organic Matcha Green Tea powder
- 4 free-range egg whites
- 1 cup free-range sour cream
- ¼ tsp cream of tartar
- 1 tsp vanilla extract
- ⅔ cup 100% pure cane sugar

Cooking Directions

1. Set oven to 250 degrees, and line baking sheets with parchment paper. Set to the side.
2. In a medium bowl, beat together egg whites and vanilla bean powder. And cream of tartar and Matcha with an electric mixer until foamy. Gradually add sugar to the mixture (1 tbsp at a time), until beating stiff peaks form and sugar dissolves.
3. Drop rounded tablespoons of mixture onto baking sheets. Allow to bake for 75 minutes or until meringues begin to brown. Turn off oven and allow meringues to sit in oven over night with oven light on or for a minimum of 8 hours.

4. When ready to serve, top each meringue with 1 tsp sour cream and one strawberry. Store leftover meringues in an airtight container.

Sweet Green Falafels

Yield: *Six Servings*

Active Time: *15 minutes*

Cooking Time: *40 minutes*

Total Time: *55 minutes*

Ingredients

- 3 tsp organic Matcha Green Tea powder
- 1 (15 ounce) can organic Garbanzo beans, drained
- 2 organic sweet potatoes
- 2 cups unbleached all-purpose flour
- 1 large free-range egg
- ½ tsp coriander
- 1 tsp ground cinnamon
- 1 tsp garlic powder
- Cooking spray

Cooking Directions

1. Set oven to 375 degrees and coat a baking sheet with cooking spray.
2. Poke sweet potatoes a few times with a fork, and place in a microwave safe dish. Cook potatoes on HIGH for 5 minutes, remove potatoes from microwave and flip over and cook for an additional 3 to 5 minutes. Remove from microwave and allow potatoes to cool before peeling and cutting potatoes into large chunks.

3. Using a potato masher or a fork mash chickpeas in a medium bowl. Mix in sweet potatoes, Matcha, and egg. Stir until mixture is smooth. Add flour, garlic powder, cumin, and coriander to the see in to the potato mixture, mix until the batter becomes thick and pasty almost like cookie dough.
4. Section dough off into 1" balls and arrange onto prepared baking sheet, and gently flatten into patties.
5. Bake for a minimum of 30 minutes flipping every 15 minutes.

Green Cream Berry Blend

Yield: Twenty-Four servings

Active Time: 10 minutes

Cooking Time: 0 minutes

Total Time: 4 hours, 50 minutes

Ingredients

- 1 cup frozen blueberries
- 1 cup frozen raspberries
- 1 (11 ounce) can organic mandarin oranges, drained
- 3 tsp organic Matcha Green Tea powder
- 2 organic frozen bananas, sliced (peel before freezing)
- 8 ounce low-fat cream cheese
- 1 ½ cup frozen no sugar whipped topping, thawed
- ½ cup 100% pure cane sugar

Cooking Directions

1. Whip cream cheese, sugar, and Matcha together in a medium bowl until the cheese becomes fluffy. Gently fold in bananas, berries, and oranges.
2. Dump mixture into 9"x13" baking dish, and cover with plastic wrap. Place dish into freezer for 4 hours to set.
3. Thaw for 30 minutes before serving.

Minty Green Shake

Yield: *Two Servings*

Active Time: *5 minutes*

Cooking Time: *0 minutes*

Total Time: *5 minutes*

Ingredients

- ½ cup frozen honeydew mellow, chopped
- 2 frozen bananas (peel before freezing)
- 1 tsp organic Matcha Green Tea powder
- ⅓ cup organic plain soy yogurt
- 1 cup organic vanilla soy milk
- 1 tbsp organic Agave nectar
- 3 drops peppermint extract
- Spring water ice (optional)

Cooking Directions

1. Add all of the ingredients to the blender, and puree until all of the ingredients become completely smooth.
2. Pour into your favorite glass and enjoy!

Matcha Waffles

Yield: *Ten Servings*

Active Time: *10 minutes*

Bake Time: *15 minutes*

Total Time: *30 minutes*

Ingredients

- 2 tsp organic Matcha Green Tea powder
- 1 ½ cup free-range buttermilk
- 2 large free-range egg, lightly beaten
- 2 cup 100% pure cane sugar
- 2 cup fresh strawberries, chopped
- 1 ¾ cups unbleached all-purpose flour
- 1 tsp aluminum-free baking powder
- 5 tbsp organic raw honey
- 3 tbsp Unrefined Extra Virgin Olive oil
- 1 ½ tsp vanilla bean powder, divided
- 1 tsp Himalayan Pink Salt
- Cooking spray

Cooking Directions

1. Combine flour, Matcha, baking powder, vanilla bean powder, salt, and sugar in a large bowl. Mix well to blend all of the dry ingredients, form a well in the center. Set to the side.
2. In a separate bowl, beat together eggs, milk, and oil. Mix well until all of the ingredients are emulsified. Pour into the center of the well in the dry ingredients bowl, and mix vigorously until the batter becomes smooth. Be sure that all lumps have been removed.

3. Lightly grease your waffle maker and add waffle mixture according to the manufacturer's instructions.
4. In the meantime, dump honey and strawberries into a small bowl and mix well to coat the strawberries. Serve syrup over the warm Matcha waffles.

Whole-Wheat Green Pancakes

Yield: *Two Servings*

Active Time: *5 minutes*

Cooking Time: *10 minutes*

Total Time: *15 minutes*

Ingredients

- 2 tsp organic Matcha Green Tea powder
- ¼ cup unbleached all-purpose flour
- ¼ cup whole-wheat flour
- 1 tbsp brown sugar
- 1 tbsp aluminum-free baking powder
- 1 free-range egg
- 6 tbsp grass-fed milk
- 1 tbsp ghee
- Nonstick cooking spray

Cooking Directions

1. In a medium bowl, stir together Matcha all-purpose flour, whole-wheat flour, sugar, and baking powder.
2. Combine egg, milk, and melted margarine in a separate bowl.
3. All he combined dry ingredients to the egg mixture. Stir until the batter becomes lumpy.
4. Lightly spray a heavy skillet or griddle with cooking spray.
5. Measure ¼ cup of pancake batter for each pancake.

6. Cook pancakes until the bubbles begin to form on top half and pancake begins to look dry. The bottoms should be golden brown.
7. Flip the pancake and allow the opposite side to brown.

Green Spinach Triangles

Yield: *Three Servings*

Active Time: *20 minutes*

Cooking Time: *30 minutes*

Total Time: *50 minutes*

Ingredients

- 4 tbsp organic Matcha Green Tea powder
- 9 ounces whole-wheat flour
- 10 ounces fresh spinach, rinsed and stems removed
- ⅜ cup medium onion, finely chopped
- 2 tbsp lemon juice, freshly squeezed
- ¾ clove garlic, finely chopped
- 1 ¼ tsp fresh basil leaves, chopped
- 1 ¼ tsp fresh mint leaves, chopped
- ⅛ tsp garlic salt
- ¼ tsp 100% pure cane sugar
- ¼ tsp organic active dry yeast
- ¼ cup warm Spring water
- 1 ¼ tsp Unrefined Extra Virgin Olive oil
- ¼ tsp Himalayan Pink Salt

Cooking Directions

1. Set oven to 450 degrees.
2. Stir together Matcha, sugar, yeast, and hot water in a small bowl and set aside. Allow bubbles to form in the yeast, and then pour in salt and olive oil.
3. In a large bowl, combine flour and yeast mixture to form into a partially, soft dough.

4. On a lightly floured surface, knead the dough with your hands using slightly heavy pressure. Continue kneading the dough until it reaches a smooth and soft texture. This process should take at least 15 minutes.
5. Place dough in a large bowl, and cover bowl with a clean towel to allow dough to rise and rest.
6. Roughly chop spinach.
7. In a large pot, add salt, water and spinach. Bring this to a boil and allow to cook for 2 minutes, or until the spinach has wilted.
8. Drain the spinach well and return to the pot. Add onions, lemon juice, garlic, basil, mint, and garlic salt to the spinach. Allow to cook until flavors are well combined or for 2 minutes.
9. Remove dough from bowl, and cut into golf-ball size pieces. Roll the pieces into 5-inch wide disks. Be sure the disks are about ¼ inch thick.
10. In the center of each "disk", dump 1 tbsp of the spinach filing.
11. After all disks have been dressed with spinach filing, fold up three sides of the disk to form into a triangle. Be sure to leave a small hole in the center to allow steam to release while baking.
12. Bake for 10 to 15 minutes, or until golden brown.

Simple Lemon Matcha Pie

Yield: *Eight Servings*

Active Time: *30 minutes*

Cooking Time: *30 minutes*

Total Time: *5 hours, 10 minutes*

Ingredients

- 2 tbsp organic Matcha Green Tea powder
- 1 ½ cups graham crackers, finely crushed (20 squares)
- ⅓ cup ghee
- 3 tbsp 100% pure cane sugar
- 4 cups vanilla ice cream
- 1 (6 ounce) can frozen lemonade concentrate, thawed
- Few drops yellow food color, if desired
- Grated lemon or lime peel

Cooking Directions

1. Set oven to 375 degrees.
2. Combine graham cracker, butter, and sugar in a medium bowl. Press graham cracker mixture firmly against bottom and side of 9"x1 ¼" pie plate.
3. Bake for about 10 minutes or until crust is light brown. Remove from oven and set aside.
4. Stir together ice cream, lemonade concentrate, Matcha, and food color in a large bowl. Spoon ice cream mixture in crust.
5. Place in freezer and allow pie to freeze for about 4 hours or until firm and set. Thaw pie for

about 5 minutes before cutting, and garnish
with grated lemon peel.   Serve immediately.

Cheesy Strata

Yield: *Twelve Servings*

Active Time: *30 minutes*

Cooking Time: *1 hour*

Total Time: *1 hour, 30 minutes*

Ingredients

- 4 tbsp organic Matcha Green Tea powder
- 10 slice stale white bread, quartered
- 8 free-range eggs, beaten
- 3 cups grass-fed Monterey Jack cheese, shredded
- 3 cups grass-fed cheddar cheese, shredded
- 2 cups grass-fed milk
- 2 cups grass-fed half-and-half
- ¼ cup ghee
- 1 tsp Worcestershire sauce
- 1 tsp brown sugar
- ¼ tsp paprika
- ⅛ tsp cayenne pepper
- ½ tsp onion powder
- 1 tsp mustard powder
- 1 tbsp fresh parsley, chopped
- Himalayan Pink Salt and pepper to taste
- Cooking spray

Cooking Directions

1. Coat a 9"x13" baking dish with cooking spray and set aside.
2. Add ghee one side of each bread quarter and layer half of the buttered bread onto the bottom

of the prepared baking dish. Top with 1 ½ cup
Monterey Jack cheese, 1 ½ cup cheddar cheese,
and remaining bread slices. Set aside.

3. Whisk together Matcha, eggs, half-and-half,
   milk, brown sugar, cayenne, onion powder,
   mustard powder, Worcestershire sauce, salt,
   and pepper in a large bowl. Pour egg mixture
   over cheese and bread. Cover baking dish with
   plastic wrap and refrigerate overnight or for at
   least 8 hours.

4. The following morning, preheat oven to 325
   degrees.

5. Remove baking dish from fridge and uncover.

6. Bake for 1 hours or until eggs are fully set and
   cheese is bubbly. Allow strata to stand for 10
   minutes before serving and garnish with fresh
   parsley.

Green Soup with Tofu

Yield: *Four servings*

Active Time: *20 minutes*

Cooking Time: *1 hour*

Total Time: *1 hour, 20 minutes*

Ingredients

- 1 ½ tsp olive oil
- ½ white onion, finely chopped
- 1 ½ cloves garlic, pressed
- 2 small red potatoes, diced
- ½ cup carrots, peeled and diced
- 8 ounces dry green split peas
- 2 cups vegetable broth
- 1 tbsp organic Matcha Green Tea powder
- 8 ounces soft tofu
- ½ (6 ounce) bag fresh spinach, finely chopped
- 1 ½ tsp dried basil
- Salt and pepper to taste

Cooking Directions

1. In a large skillet, heat olive oil over medium heat. Add garlic and onion, and sauté for at least 5 minutes or until tender. Remove from heat and set aside.
2. Add sautéed onion and garlic, potatoes, carrots, split peas, and vegetable broth to a large pot. Bring to a boil over medium- high heat.
3. Reduce heat to low and allow to simmer for at least 60 minutes.

4. In the meantime, using a blender or a food processor, Matcha puree tofu and spinach, and add to pot.
5. Serve hot, and enjoy!

Chapter 4 – Natural Deodorants

Nasty chemicals and toxins like propylene glycol, phthalates, and parabens are found in many of the skin care and hair care products that are falling off of the store shelves today. Unfortunately, many people that use them are unaware of the potential health problems and risks that many of these products can cause.

The best way to fight and protect yourself against these harmful products and chemicals is to make your own. Homemade deodorants, hair care, and skin care products are some of the easiest and fun beauty products that you can make from the total comfort of your home. This book provides you with valuable information and recipes on how you can make the BEST skin care, deodorants, and hair care products by using Matcha green tea powder along with a variety of inexpensive organic products.

Tips

- To increase your homemade deodorant's shelf life, you should place in the fridge after each use.
- Strive to use all organic ingredients. This will decrease the risk of toxins and harmful chemicals entering your body through one of the most sensitive areas on your body.
- Always apply these deodorants about 5 minutes before putting on clothes. The deodorant should be completely dry and absorbed to prevent stains forming in clothes.

- All measurements are suggestions. You go as heavy as you want to on these ingredients. Be easy on the Matcha green tea, you don't want to have GREEN armpits. However, it's completely up to you!
- Date and label your deodorants to ensure proper safety.

These are some of the best recipes for natural armpit odor control using Matcha Green Tea powder. These healthy deodorants will work their supernatural powers on you long after your first application. Since chlorophyll is a natural deodorant, you will be able to stay a lot fresher than you think. The more you use these deodorants the less you will be dependent on those highly toxic, disgusting, chemical infested deodorants. No antiperspirant chemicals needed.

Incorporating these deodorants into your regimen will not only give you healthy and beautiful skin, but you feel better. These deodorants take outer nutrition to another level! You'll love the feel and the pores under your armpits won't get clogged.

Natural Green Cream Baking Soda Deodorant

Ingredients

- 1 tsp organic Matcha Green Tea powder
- 4 drops Tea Tree Oil
- 3 drops Lemongrass Oil
- 2 drops Peppermint Oil
- 5 tbsp Unrefined Virgin Coconut Oil
- ¼ cup aluminum-free baking soda
- ¼ tbsp cornstarch

Directions

1. Mix together all ingredients in a small, sterilized mason jar using a Bamboo stick.
2. Allow the deodorant to fuse for a minimum of 30 minutes before using.
3. Smear a small quantity of the deodorant under your arms, and feel the difference.

Very Green and Very Basic Deodorant

Ingredients

- 1 tsp organic Matcha Green Tea powder
- ½ cup Unrefined Virgin Coconut Oil
- 3 tbsp Epsom Salt

Directions

1. Mix together all ingredients in a small, sterilized mason jar using a Bamboo stick.
2. Allow the deodorant to fuse for a minimum of 30 minutes before using.
3. Smear a small quantity of the deodorant under your arms, and feel the difference.

Mean Green Eucalyptus

Ingredients

- 8 drops eucalyptus oil
- 1 tsp organic Matcha Green Tea powder
- 12 drops tea tree oil
- ¼ cup aluminum-free baking soda
- ¼ cup arrowroot powder
- 4 tbsp Unrefined Virgin Coconut Oil

Directions

1. Mix together all ingredients in a small, sterilized mason jar using a Bamboo stick.
2. Allow the deodorant to fuse for a minimum of 30 minutes before using.
3. Smear a small quantity of the deodorant under your arms, and feel the difference.

Matcha Orange Spice Cake

Ingredients

- 10 drops sweet orange oil
- 1 tsp organic Matcha Green Tea powder
- 10 drops cinnamon oil
- 2 tbsp Unrefined Virgin Coconut Oil
- ⅓ cup aluminum-free baking soda
- ⅓ cup arrowroot powder

Directions

1. Mix together all ingredients in a small, sterilized mason jar using a Bamboo stick.
2. Allow the deodorant to fuse for a minimum of 30 minutes before using.
3. Smear a small quantity of the deodorant under your arms, and feel the difference.

Minty Fresh

Ingredients

- 20 drops peppermint oil
- 1 tsp organic Matcha Green Tea powder
- 1 tbsp Unrefined Virgin Coconut Oil
- 3 tbsp raw cocoa butter
- 3 tsp Aloe Vera gel
- 1 tbsp aluminum-free baking soda
- 2 tbsp cornstarch

Directions

1. Boil some water in a small pot, and place a small Mason jar in the pot. Lid removed. Boil the jar for a minimum of 5 minutes, drop in the cocoa butter and coconut oil into the Mason jar. Allow to melt, stirring frequently with a Bamboo stick.
2. Carefully remove the jar from the pot using a pair of tongs. Slowly stir in baking soda, Matcha, cornstarch, Aloe Vera gel, and peppermint oil.
3. Allow the ingredients to fuse for about 30 minutes before using.
4. Smear a small quantity of the deodorant under your arms, and feel the difference.

Grape & Matcha

Ingredients

- 2 tbsp Shea Butter
- 2 tbsp raw cocoa butter
- 2 tbsp arrowroot powder
- ½ tbsp aluminum-free baking soda
- 1 tsp organic Matcha Green Tea powder
- 10 drops nutmeg oil
- 10 drops grapefruit oil
- 10 drops lavender oil
- 3 drops Vitamin E oil

Directions

1. Boil some water in a small pot, and place a small Mason jar in the pot. Lid removed. Boil the jar for a minimum of 5 minutes, drop in the cocoa butter and shea butter into the Mason jar. Allow to melt, stirring frequently with a Bamboo stick.
2. Carefully remove the jar from the pot using a pair of tongs. Slowly stir in remaining ingredients.
3. Allow the ingredients to fuse for about 30 minutes before using.
4. Smear a small quantity of the deodorant under your arms, and feel the difference.

Vetiver Green

Ingredients

- 1 tsp organic Matcha Green Tea powder
- 15 drops rose oil
- 10 drops vetiver oil
- 15 drops lime oil
- ⅛ cup rose water

Directions

1. Pour all ingredients into the spray bottle. Cover with mister and shake well. Set aside and allow the ingredients to fuse for a minimum of 30 minutes before using.
2. Spray under your arms and enjoy the freshness!

Minty Fresh Matcha

Ingredients

- 10 drops lemongrass oil
- 1 tsp organic Matcha Green Tea powder
- 3 drops peppermint oil
- 2 tbsp arrowroot powder
- 2 tbsp aluminum-free baking soda

Directions

1. Mix together all ingredients in a small, sterilized mason jar using a Bamboo stick.
2. Allow the deodorant to fuse for a minimum of 30 minutes before using.
3. Smear a small quantity of the deodorant under your arms, and feel the difference.

Matcha Man

Ingredients

- 6 drops Cedar wood oil
- 1 tsp organic Matcha Green Tea powder
- 5 drops tea tree oil
- 4 tbsp Unrefined Virgin Coconut oil
- ¼ cup cornstarch
- ¼ cup aluminum-free baking soda

Directions

Mix together all ingredients in a small, sterilized mason jar using a Bamboo stick.

Allow the deodorant to fuse for a minimum of 30 minutes before using.

Smear a small quantity of the deodorant under your arms, and feel the difference.

Green Island Breeze

Ingredients

- 1 tsp organic Matcha Green Tea powder
- 2 tbsp Unrefined Virgin Coconut oil
- 5 drops grapefruit oil
- 3 drops peppermint oil
- 3 drops sweet orange oil
- 3 drops lemongrass oil
- ¼ cup arrowroot powder
- ¼ cup aluminum-free baking soda

Directions

1. Mix together all ingredients in a small, sterilized mason jar using a Bamboo stick.
2. Allow the deodorant to fuse for a minimum of 30 minutes before using.
3. Smear a small quantity of the deodorant under your arms, and feel the difference.

Matcha Musk

Ingredients

- 1 tsp organic Matcha Green Tea powder
- 10 drops pine oil
- 10 drops tea tree oil
- 10 juniper oil
- 5 drops myrrh oil
- 1 tbsp Unrefined Virgin Coconut oil
- ½ raw cocoa butter
- 1 ½ tbsp beeswax

Directions

1. Boil some water in a small pot, and place a small Mason jar in the pot. Lid removed. Boil the jar for a minimum of 5 minutes, drop in the cocoa butter and beeswax into the Mason jar. Allow to melt, stirring frequently with a Bamboo stick.
2. Carefully remove the jar from the pot using a pair of tongs. Slowly stir in remaining ingredients.
3. Allow the ingredients to fuse for about 30 minutes before using.
4. Smear a small quantity of the deodorant under your arms, and feel the difference.

Extra-Strength Matcha Musk

Ingredients

- 1 tsp organic Matcha Green Tea powder
- 5 drops frankincense oil
- 10 drops cypress oil
- 10 drops vanilla oil
- 15 drops sandalwood oil
- 1 tbsp Unrefined Virgin Coconut oil
- ½ tbsp raw cocoa butter
- 1 ½ tbsp beeswax

Directions

1. Boil some water in a small pot, and place a small Mason jar in the pot. Lid removed. Boil the jar for a minimum of 5 minutes, drop in the cocoa butter and coconut oil into the Mason jar. Allow to melt, stirring frequently with a Bamboo stick.
2. Carefully remove the jar from the pot using a pair of tongs. Slowly stir in remaining ingredients.
3. Allow the ingredients to fuse for about 30 minutes before using.
4. Smear a small quantity of the deodorant under your arms, and feel the difference.

Chapter 5 – Natural Skin and Hair Care Recipes

Green Matcha Mask

Ingredients

- 1 tsp organic Matcha Green Tea powder
- ½ tsp Unrefined Virgin Coconut oil
- Spring Water

Directions

1. Mix together one tablespoon of Matcha Green Tea Powder in a small bowl and add ½ tablespoon of coconut oil and small amount of water.
2. Stir using a Bamboo spoon while slowly adding. Continue this to until the mixture becomes a smooth paste. Be sure the mixture does not become too runny.
3. Apply the mask to your face and neck. Allow to sit for at least an hour or longer.

Black Matcha Acne Magnet

Ingredients

- 1 tsp organic Matcha Green Tea powder
- 4 tsp activated black charcoal powder
- 2 tbsp Bentonite Green clay
- ½ cup cornstarch
- ½ tsp Unrefined Virgin Coconut oil
- Spring Water

Directions

1. Mix together one tablespoon of Matcha Green Tea Powder in a small bowl and add ½ tablespoon of coconut oil and small amount of water.
2. Stir using a Bamboo spoon while slowly adding. Continue this to until the mixture becomes a smooth paste. Be sure the mixture does not become too runny.
3. Apply the mask to your face and neck. Allow to sit for at least an hour or longer.

Green Matcha Moisturizer

Ingredients

- 1 tsp organic Matcha Green Tea powder
- 1 ½ cups almond oil
- ½ cup raw coco butter
- 3 tbsp Aloe Vera
- 8 tbsp beeswax, grated and melted
- 4 tbsp green tea leaves
- 10 drops lemongrass oil
- 2 cup hot Spring Water

Directions

1. Seep tea leaves in hot water for about 5 minutes. Remove the tea leaves and allow the tea to cool.
2. Blend together almond oil, lemongrass oil, Matcha, beeswax, and Aloe Vera in an immersion blender.
3. Dump mixture into your favorite glass jar, and use at your desire.

Matcha Green Tea Body Scrub

Ingredients

- 1 cup 100% pure cane sugar
- 1 tsp organic Matcha Green Tea powder
- ½ cup Unrefined Virgin Coconut oil
- 1 tbsp green tea leaves

Directions

1. Mix together all ingredients in a large bowl using a Bamboo spoon, and pour into your favorite Mason jar or glass jar.
2. Use whenever you're ready!

Matcha Green Toner

Ingredients

- 6 drops Sandalwood oil
- 3 drops thyme oil
- 1 tbsp organic unpasteurized apple cider vinegar
- ½ cup boiling Spring water
- 1 tsp organic Matcha Green Tea powder
- 1 tbsp green tea leaves

Directions

1. Add green tea leaves into a medium bowl and pour boiling water into the bowl. Allow to seep for about one hour and strain.
2. Add Matcha, Sandalwood oil, thyme oil, vinegar, and about 7 tablespoons of green tea to a 4 ounce spray bottle.
3. Label, date, and place in fridge to cool and mingle overnight.
4. Mist on face at night before bed!

Matcha Green Lemon Hair Rinse

Ingredients

- 20 drops lemongrass oil
- 1 cup Spring water
- 3 tbsp green tea leaves
- 1 lemon, freshly grated and juiced

Directions

1. Add lemon zest and spring water to medium pot and bring to a boil. Dump in green tea leaves. Remove from heat and strain.
2. Once cooled pour into your favorite spray bottle and spritz on your hair each morning and night.

Conclusion

Well, that's all! You have been given some of the BEST information on Matcha green tea! How far you go on your journey with Matcha green tea is totally up to you. Taking the first step is always the hardest, even when it comes to bettering your health. However, the decision to add Matcha green tea to your lifestyle will give your body no choice but to thank you for it.

Be aware that your body will begin to detox more effectively once you begin consuming and using Matcha green tea. This means that you may have some reactions that are not deadly, but are a result of your body becoming more efficient in the daily detoxification process. However, in the long-term you will be happy that you decided to make the change.

Hopefully, you will enjoy and appreciate the process and become accustomed to using deodorants that are free from deadly and unhealthy ingredients. Fight for your health, and always go the organic route.

Thanks you for reading!

I hope you enjoyed this Ebook on Matcha green tea. If you did I would greatly appreciate if you left a review. Follow my Amazon author page for updates on my latest books or send me an email directly at:

A_hunter2015@hotmail.com

www.ingramcontent.com/pod-product-compliance
Lightning Source LLC
Chambersburg PA
CBHW070940180526
45168CB00003B/1117